LOW OXALATE FOOD LIST

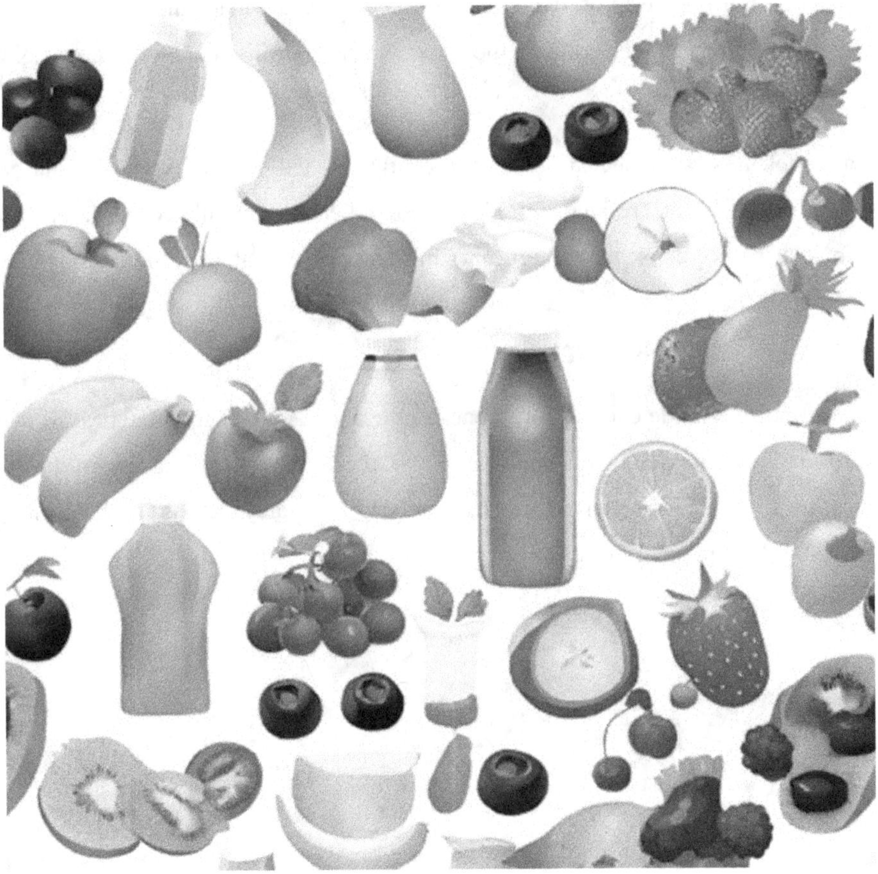

LYSANDRA QUINN

TABLE OF CONTENTS

INTRODUCTION

In the dimly lit cafe of a quaint coastal town, I found myself engrossed in a conversation that would change the course of my career and, ultimately, the lives of countless individuals seeking relief from an invisible, excruciating enemy: oxalates. As a seasoned dietitian, I thought I had encountered every dietary challenge under the sun. But it was on that fateful day, over a cup of steaming chamomile tea, that my journey into the world of oxalates began.

Picture this: a brisk autumn evening, the air crisp with the scent of saltwater and fallen leaves, and the gentle hum of conversation around me. I was enjoying my usual spot near the window, taking in the serene view of the ocean waves crashing against the shore. The cafe, known for its array of pastries and aromatic coffees, was my haven, a place where I gathered my thoughts and immersed myself in the world of nutrition.

As I sipped my tea, I noticed a young woman sitting at the corner table. Her name was Amelia, and she had been a regular at the cafe for months, always accompanied by a worn-out notebook filled with scribbles and diagrams. There was an air of determination about her, an unmistakable energy that intrigued me. I couldn't help but be drawn to her, my curiosity piqued by her unwavering focus.

One evening, as we both sat in our usual spots, fate brought us together. Amelia's notebook fell to the floor, and I rushed to help her pick up her scattered notes. It was then that I glimpsed a glimpse of the revelations hidden within her pages. Graphs, tables, and meticulously recorded food items—everything was related to oxalates. The word "oxalate" was written everywhere, almost like a secret code that only she seemed to understand.

With a gracious smile, she thanked me for my assistance and introduced herself. In the following minutes, Amelia began to unravel her story, one that would captivate me and lead me down a path I could have never anticipated.

Amelia, an athletic and vibrant woman in her late twenties, had been suffering from chronic pain for years. She had consulted numerous doctors, undergone a battery of tests, and tried various medications to no avail. The pain that gripped her was so severe that it had become her constant companion, stealing away the joy from her life and imprisoning her in a never-ending cycle of agony.

One day, in the depths of her despair, Amelia stumbled upon an article about oxalates and their potential role in chronic pain. Intrigued, she began her own research journey, educating herself on the intricacies of these tiny, often overlooked crystals. She meticulously tracked her dietary choices, jotting down every morsel that entered her body, and she noticed a pattern emerging. It became clear that certain foods triggered her pain, while others offered her relief.

The moment of revelation for Amelia was both transformative and terrifying. She realized that oxalates, compounds naturally found in many common foods, were the culprits behind her anguish. Her diet, once thought to be healthy, was unknowingly contributing to her suffering. As she delved deeper into the world of low oxalate foods, she experienced moments of respite, and her pain began to ebb away, like a receding tide.

Listening to Amelia's story, I was awestruck by her determination and the profound impact that a simple change in diet had made on her life. It was a wake-up call that transcended the confines of that cafe, leaving an indelible mark on my soul. I knew in that moment that my purpose as a female dietitian was about to take an unexpected and powerful turn.

Our journey together had just begun. I embarked on a quest to unravel the intricacies of oxalates, researching the latest scientific literature and collaborating with experts in the field. I was determined to understand how oxalates impacted our bodies, why they could be both friend and foe, and most importantly, how we could harness this knowledge to empower individuals like Amelia to regain control over their lives.

Low Oxalate Food List is the culmination of our shared journey, a testament to the power of knowledge and the unyielding spirit of those who refuse to be defeated by chronic pain. Within the pages of this book, you will find not just a list of low oxalate foods, but a comprehensive guide to understanding oxalates, managing your diet, and regaining the freedom to live a life unburdened by pain.

We will delve deep into the science behind oxalates, exploring the mechanisms by which they affect our bodies and learning why some individuals are more susceptible to their harmful effects. You will discover the hidden sources of oxalates in everyday foods, uncover the surprising culprits lurking in your kitchen, and gain the tools you need to make informed dietary choices.

The journey ahead is both enlightening and empowering, as we explore the vast array of low oxalate foods that can be incorporated into your daily meals. You will find delectable recipes, meal plans, and practical tips to help you transition to a low oxalate diet without sacrificing taste or variety.

But this book is more than just a manual for managing oxalate intake. It is a testament to the resilience of the human spirit, the unyielding determination to overcome obstacles, and the boundless potential of the human body to heal when given the right tools. Amelia's story, my journey, and the stories of countless others who have triumphed over oxalates will inspire you to embark on your own path to healing.

Whether you are a chronic pain sufferer seeking relief, a curious reader eager to learn about the hidden world of oxalates, or a dedicated healthcare professional looking for tools to better serve your patients, Low Oxalate Food List is your guide to a transformative journey.

Join us as we explore the fascinating realm of oxalates, unveil the secrets of low oxalate eating, and embark on a path toward a healthier, pain-free future. Together, we will uncover the power of informed dietary choices and rewrite the stories of our lives, one meal at a time.

CHAPTER 1

What is Oxalate?

Oxalate is a natural compound found in many foods and produced by the human body as a waste product of metabolism. It plays a role in the formation of kidney stones, as well as contributing to the development of other health issues, when it accumulates in excessive amounts in the body.

The Importance of a Low Oxalate Diet:

A low oxalate diet is recommended for individuals who are prone to kidney stones or those with certain medical conditions that can lead to oxalate buildup in the body. The importance of a low oxalate diet lies in reducing the risk of kidney stone formation and managing related health issues. Here are some key reasons why a low oxalate diet is important:

Kidney Stone Prevention: High levels of oxalate in the urine can combine with calcium to form kidney stones, which can be extremely painful and require medical intervention. By reducing oxalate intake, individuals can lower their risk of stone formation.

Management of Oxalosis: Some rare genetic disorders, such as primary hyperoxaluria, cause the excessive production of oxalate in the body. In such cases, a low oxalate diet is crucial to prevent oxalate buildup and related health complications.

Gastrointestinal Conditions: People with certain gastrointestinal disorders, such as inflammatory bowel disease or celiac disease, may be more susceptible to oxalate absorption from their diet. A low oxalate diet can help manage these conditions.

Improved Nutrient Absorption: High oxalate foods can interfere with the absorption of essential nutrients like calcium and magnesium. A low oxalate diet can help individuals ensure they are getting the full benefit of these nutrients.

Who Should Follow a Low Oxalate Diet?

Individuals who should consider following a low oxalate diet include:

Those with a History of Kidney Stones: People who have previously experienced kidney stones are at a higher risk of developing them again, and a low oxalate diet can help prevent recurrence.

Individuals with Hyperoxaluria: Those diagnosed with primary hyperoxaluria or other disorders that cause excessive oxalate production should adhere to a strict low oxalate diet under medical supervision.

People with Gastrointestinal Disorders: Those with gastrointestinal conditions that affect nutrient absorption, like Crohn's disease or celiac disease, may benefit from a low oxalate diet.

Anyone at Risk: If you have a family history of kidney stones or other risk factors for oxalate-related health issues, it's advisable to consult with a healthcare professional and consider a low oxalate diet.

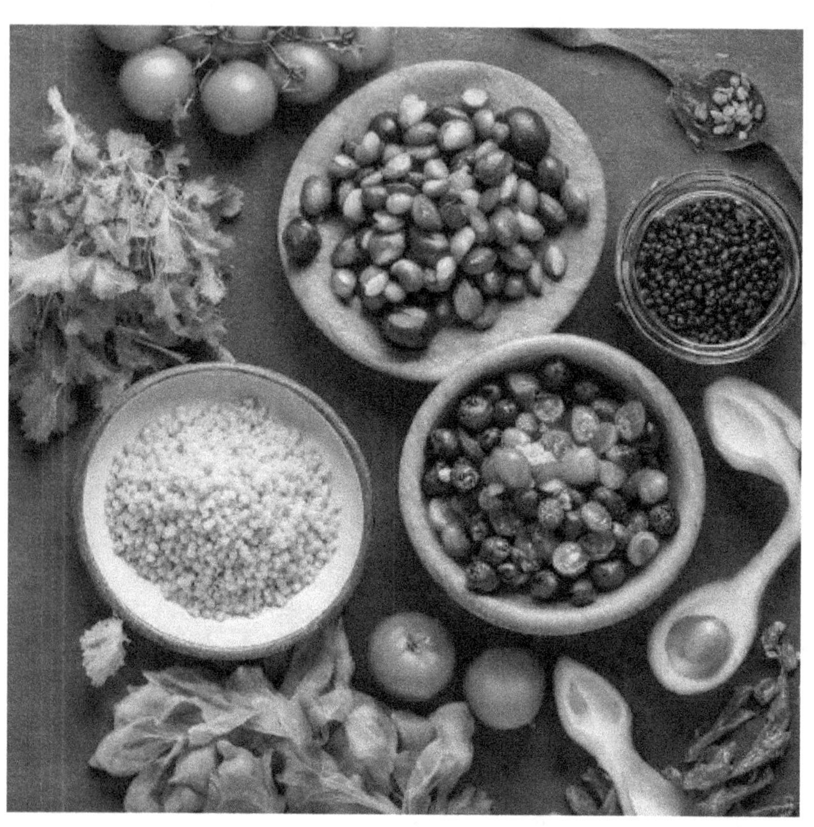

CHAPTER 2

Low Oxalate Food Categories

Vegetables

Cucumber

Oxalate content: Very low

Nutritional information (per 100g):

- Calories: 15
- Carbohydrates: 3.6g
- Fiber: 0.5g
- Vitamin K: 16.4µg
- Vitamin C: 2.8mg

Zucchini (Courgette):

Oxalate content: Low

Nutritional information (per 100g):

- Calories: 17
- Carbohydrates: 3.1g
- Fiber: 1.0g
- Vitamin K: 4.3µg
- Vitamin C: 17.9mg

Bell Peppers (Red, Green, or Yellow)

Oxalate content: Low

Nutritional information (per 100g):

- Calories: 31
- Carbohydrates: 6.0g
- Fiber: 2.1g
- Vitamin K: 7.4µg
- Vitamin C: 127.7mg

Cabbage

Oxalate content: Low

Nutritional information (per 100g):

- Calories: 25
- Carbohydrates: 5.8g
- Fiber: 2.5g
- Vitamin K: 76.0µg
- Vitamin C: 36.6mg

Celery

Oxalate content: Low

Nutritional information (per 100g):

- Calories: 16
- Carbohydrates: 3.0g
- Fiber: 1.6g
- Vitamin K: 29.3µg
- Vitamin C: 3.1mg

Asparagus

Oxalate content: Low

Nutritional information (per 100g):

- Calories: 20
- Carbohydrates: 3.7g
- Fiber: 2.0g
- Vitamin K: 41.6µg
- Vitamin C: 5.6mg

Broccoli

Oxalate content: Low

Nutritional information (per 100g):

- Calories: 55
- Carbohydrates: 11.2g
- Fiber: 2.6g
- Vitamin K: 101.6µg
- Vitamin C: 89.2mg

Cauliflower

Oxalate content: Low

Nutritional information (per 100g):

- Calories: 25
- Carbohydrates: 5.3g
- Fiber: 2.0g
- Vitamin K: 15.5µg
- Vitamin C: 48.2mg

Lettuce (Romaine or Iceberg):

Oxalate content: Low

Nutritional information (per 100g):

- Calories: 5
- Carbohydrates: 1.0g
- Fiber: 1.2g
- Vitamin K: 48.2µg
- Vitamin C: 2.8mg

Green Beans

Oxalate content: Low

Nutritional information (per 100g):

- Calories: 31
- Carbohydrates: 7.1g
- Fiber: 3.4g
- Vitamin K: 14.4µg
- Vitamin C: 16.3mg

Fruits

Blueberries

Oxalate content: Low

Nutritional information (per 100g):

- Calories: 32
- Carbohydrates: 9.7g
- Fiber: 2.4g
- Vitamin C: 9.7mg
- Vitamin K: 19.3µg

Pears

Oxalate content: Low

Nutritional information (per 100g):

- Calories: 57
- Carbohydrates: 15.5g
- Fiber: 3.1g
- Vitamin C: 3.1mg
- Vitamin K: 4.4µg

Papaya

Oxalate content: Low

Nutritional information (per 100g):

- Calories: 43
- Carbohydrates: 11.0g
- Fiber: 1.7g
- Vitamin C: 60.9mg
- Vitamin K: 2.6μg

Apples

Oxalate content: Low

Nutritional information (per 100g):

- Calories: 52
- Carbohydrates: 14.0g
- Fiber: 2.4g
- Vitamin C: 0.5mg
- Vitamin K: 2.2µg

Mango

Oxalate content: Low

- Nutritional information (per 100g):
- Calories: 60
- Carbohydrates: 15.0g
- Fiber: 1.6g
- Vitamin C: 36.4mg
- Vitamin K: 4.2µg

Watermelon:

Oxalate content: Low

Nutritional information (per 100g):

- Calories: 30
- Carbohydrates: 7.6g
- Fiber: 0.4g
- Vitamin C: 8.1mg
- Vitamin K: 0.1µg

Kiwi

Oxalate content: Low

Nutritional information (per 100g):

- Calories: 61
- Carbohydrates: 14.6g
- Fiber: 3.0g
- Vitamin C: 92.7mg
- Vitamin K: 40.3µg

Honeydew Melon:

Oxalate content: Low

Nutritional information (per 100g):

- Calories: 36
- Carbohydrates: 9.1g
- Fiber: 0.8g
- Vitamin C: 18.0mg
- Vitamin K: 1.4µg

Grapes

Oxalate content: Low

Nutritional information (per 100g):

- Calories: 69
- Carbohydrates: 18.0g
- Fiber: 0.9g
- Vitamin C: 2.3mg
- Vitamin K: 14.6µg

Cantaloupe

Oxalate content: Low

Nutritional information (per 100g):

- Calories: 34
- Carbohydrates: 8.2g
- Fiber: 0.9g
- Vitamin C: 36.7mg
- Vitamin K: 2.5µg

Grains

White Rice

Oxalate content: Low

Nutritional information (per 100g, cooked):

- Calories: 130
- Carbohydrates: 28.7g
- Fiber: 0.3g
- Protein: 2.7g

Quinoa

Oxalate content: Low

Nutritional information (per 100g, cooked):

- Calories: 120
- Carbohydrates: 21.3g
- Fiber: 2.8g
- Protein: 4.1g

Buckwheat

Oxalate content: Low

Nutritional information (per 100g, cooked):

- Calories: 92
- Carbohydrates: 19.9g
- Fiber: 2.7g
- Protein: 3.4g

Oats

Oxalate content: Low

Nutritional information (per 100g, cooked):

- Calories: 71
- Carbohydrates: 12.3g
- Fiber: 1.7g
- Protein: 2.5g

Barley

Oxalate content: Low

Nutritional information (per 100g, cooked):

- Calories: 96
- Carbohydrates: 22.9g
- Fiber: 2.0g
- Protein: 2.0g

Amaranth

Oxalate content: Low

Nutritional information (per 100g, cooked):

- Calories: 102
- Carbohydrates: 19.7g
- Fiber: 1.6g
- Protein: 3.8g

Millet

Oxalate content: Low

Nutritional information (per 100g, cooked):

- Calories: 119
- Carbohydrates: 23.7g
- Fiber: 1.3g
- Protein: 3.5g

Sorghum

Oxalate content: Low

Nutritional information (per 100g, cooked):

- Calories: 101
- Carbohydrates: 24.6g
- Fiber: 1.6g
- Protein: 3.3g

Rye

Oxalate content: Low

Nutritional information (per 100g, cooked):

- Calories: 68
- Carbohydrates: 15.1g
- Fiber: 1.6g
- Protein: 1.5g

Corn (Maize)

Oxalate content: Low

Nutritional information (per 100g, cooked):

- Calories: 96
- Carbohydrates: 21.3g
- Fiber: 2.4g
- Protein: 3.4g

Proteins

Chicken Breast

Oxalate content: Low

Nutritional information (per 100g, cooked):

- Calories: 165
- Protein: 31g
- Fat: 3.6g
- Carbohydrates: 0g

Turkey

Oxalate content: Low

Nutritional information (per 100g, cooked):

- Calories: 135
- Protein: 29g
- Fat: 1g
- Carbohydrates: 0g

Salmon

Oxalate content: Low

Nutritional information (per 100g, cooked):

- Calories: 206
- Protein: 22g
- Fat: 13.4g
- Carbohydrates: 0g

Cod (Whitefish)

Oxalate content: Low

Nutritional information (per 100g, cooked):

- Calories: 82
- Protein: 18.5g
- Fat: 0.7g
- Carbohydrates: 0g

Tofu

Oxalate content: Low

Nutritional information (per 100g, firm)

- Calories: 144
- Protein: 15.8g
- Fat: 8g
- Carbohydrates: 3.9g

Eggs

Oxalate content: Low

Nutritional information (per 100g, boiled):

- Calories: 143
- Protein: 12.6g
- Fat: 9.7g
- Carbohydrates: 0.6g

Pork Tenderloin

Oxalate content: Low

Nutritional information (per 100g, cooked):

- Calories: 143
- Protein: 29g
- Fat: 2.7g
- Carbohydrates: 0g

Lamb

Oxalate content: Low

Nutritional information (per 100g, cooked):

- Calories: 258
- Protein: 25g
- Fat: 17g
- Carbohydrates: 0g

Lean Ground Beef

Oxalate content: Low

Nutritional information (per 100g, cooked):

- Calories: 250
- Protein: 26g
- Fat: 17g
- Carbohydrates: 0g

Shrimp

Oxalate content: Low

Nutritional information (per 100g, cooked):

- Calories: 99
- Protein: 24g
- Fat: 0.3g
- Carbohydrates: 0g

Low Oxalate Dairy Products

Milk (Cow's Milk)

Oxalate content: Low

Nutritional information (per 1 cup, whole milk):

- Calories: 149
- Protein: 7.7g
- Fat: 7.9g
- Carbohydrates: 11.7g
- Calcium: 276mg

Goat's Milk:

Oxalate content: Low

Nutritional information (per 1 cup, whole milk):

- Calories: 168
- Protein: 8.7g
- Fat: 10.1g
- Carbohydrates: 10.9g
- Calcium: 327mg

Yogurt (Plain, Whole Milk):

Oxalate content: Low

Nutritional information (per 1 cup):

- Calories: 149
- Protein: 8.5g
- Fat: 7.6g
- Carbohydrates: 11.4g
- Calcium: 275mg

Low Oxalate Dairy Alternatives

Almond Milk (Unsweetened):

Oxalate content: Low

Nutritional information (per 1 cup):

- Calories: 13
- Protein: 1g
- Fat: 1g
- Carbohydrates: 0g
- Calcium: 516mg (fortified)

Coconut Milk (Unsweetened):

Oxalate content: Low

Nutritional information (per 1 cup):

Calories: 50

Protein: 0g

Fat: 4.5g

Carbohydrates: 1g

Calcium: 481mg (fortified)

Rice Milk (Unsweetened):

Oxalate content: Low

Nutritional information (per 1 cup):

- Calories: 120
- Protein: 1g
- Fat: 2.5g
- Carbohydrates: 23g
- Calcium: 316mg (fortified)

Hemp Milk (Unsweetened):

Oxalate content: Low

Nutritional information (per 1 cup):

- Calories: 70
- Protein: 2g
- Fat: 6g
- Carbohydrates: 1g
- Calcium: 300mg (fortified)

Cashew Milk (Unsweetened):

Oxalate content: Low

Nutritional information (per 1 cup):

Calories: 25

Protein: 0g

Fat: 2.5g

Carbohydrates: 1g

Calcium: 450mg (fortified)

Soy Milk (Unsweetened):

Oxalate content: Low

Nutritional information (per 1 cup):

- Calories: 80
- Protein: 7g
- Fat: 4g
- Carbohydrates: 4g
- Calcium: 300mg (fortified)

Oat Milk (Unsweetened):

Oxalate content: Low

Nutritional information (per 1 cup):

- Calories: 80
- Protein: 1g
- Fat: 1.5g
- Carbohydrates: 16g
- Calcium: 350mg (fortified)

CHAPTER 3

High Oxalate Foods to Avoid

Spinach

Oxalate content: High

Nutritional information (per 100g, raw):

- Calories: 23
- Carbohydrates: 3.6g
- Fiber: 2.2g
- Calcium: 99mg
- Vitamin C: 47.9mg

Rhubarb

Oxalate content: Very high

Nutritional information (per 100g, raw):

- Calories: 21
- Carbohydrates: 4.5g
- Fiber: 1.8g
- Calcium: 86mg
- Vitamin C: 8.2mg

Beet Greens

Oxalate content: High

Nutritional information (per 100g, cooked):

- Calories: 22
- Carbohydrates: 4.3g
- Fiber: 3.7g
- Calcium: 117mg
- Vitamin C: 30.0mg

Swiss Chard

Oxalate content: High

Nutritional information (per 100g, cooked):

- Calories: 19
- Carbohydrates: 3.7g
- Fiber: 2.0g
- Calcium: 51mg
- Vitamin C: 18.0mg

Spinach Pasta

Oxalate content: High

Nutritional information (per 100g, cooked):

- Calories: 159
- Carbohydrates: 32.8g
- Fiber: 1.5g
- Calcium: 21mg

Okra

Oxalate content: High

Nutritional information (per 100g, cooked):

- Calories: 33
- Carbohydrates: 7.5g
- Fiber: 3.2g
- Calcium: 77mg
- Vitamin C: 21.1mg

Almonds

Oxalate content: High

Nutritional information (per 100g):

- Calories: 576
- Carbohydrates: 21.7g
- Fiber: 12.5g
- Calcium: 264mg
- Vitamin C: 0mg

Cashews

Oxalate content: High

Nutritional information (per 100g):

- Calories: 553

- Carbohydrates: 30.2g

- Fiber: 3.3g

- Calcium: 37mg

- Vitamin C: 0.5mg

Peanuts

Oxalate content: High

Nutritional information (per 100g):

- Calories: 567
- Carbohydrates: 16.1g
- Fiber: 8.5g
- Calcium: 76mg
- Vitamin C: 0mg

Chocolate

Oxalate content: High

Nutritional information (per 100g):

- Calories: 546
- Carbohydrates: 60.5g
- Fiber: 7.1g
- Calcium: 73mg
- Vitamin C: 0.8mg

Tea (Black and Herbal)

Oxalate content: High

Nutritional information (per 8 oz cup):

- Calories: 2
- Carbohydrates: 0.5g
- Fiber: 0g
- Calcium: 3-10mg
- Vitamin C: 0mg

Potatoes (baked with skin)

Oxalate content: High

Nutritional information (per 100g, baked with skin):

- Calories: 93
- Carbohydrates: 21.2g
- Fiber: 2.2g
- Calcium: 17mg
- Vitamin C: 19.7mg

Berries (Blackberries and Raspberries)

Oxalate content: High

Nutritional information (per 100g):

- Calories: Varies
- Carbohydrates: Varies
- Fiber: Varies
- Calcium: Varies
- Vitamin C: Varies

Grapes (Red and Green)

Oxalate content: High

Nutritional information (per 100g):

- Calories: 69
- Carbohydrates: 18g
- Fiber: 0.9g
- Calcium: 10mg
- Vitamin C: 3.2mg

Figs

Oxalate content: High

Nutritional information (per 100g, dried):

- Calories: 249
- Carbohydrates: 63.9g
- Fiber: 9.8g
- Calcium: 162mg
- Vitamin C: 1.2mg

Beets

Oxalate content: High

Nutritional information (per 100g, cooked):

- Calories: 43
- Carbohydrates: 9.6g
- Fiber: 2.8g
- Calcium: 16mg
- Vitamin C: 4.9mg

Soy Products (Soybeans and Tofu):

Oxalate content: High

Nutritional information (per 100g, cooked tofu):

- Calories: 145
- Carbohydrates: 1.6g
- Fiber: 0.9g
- Calcium: 350mg
- Vitamin C: 0mg

Nuts (Walnuts and Pecans):

Oxalate content: High

Nutritional information (per 100g):

- Calories: Varies
- Carbohydrates: Varies
- Fiber: Varies
- Calcium: Varies
- Vitamin C: 0mg

Lentils

Oxalate content: High

Nutritional information (per 100g, cooked):

- Calories: 116
- Carbohydrates: 20g
- Fiber: 7.9g
- Calcium: 19mg
- Vitamin C: 3.5mg

Black Tea

Oxalate content: High

Nutritional information (per 8 oz cup):

- Calories: 2
- Carbohydrates: 0.5g
- Fiber: 0g
- Calcium: 2-10mg
- Vitamin C: 0mg

CONCLUSION

In the pages of "Low Oxalate Food List," we have embarked on a journey of discovery, empowerment, and transformation. From the moment my path intersected with the remarkable Amelia, we've unveiled the intricate world of oxalates and their profound impact on our lives.

As a dedicated female dietitian, I have witnessed the power of knowledge, the strength of informed choices, and the remarkable resilience of the human spirit. Our quest to understand oxalates, from their effects on the body to the practical steps for managing their intake, has led us to this pivotal moment.

The information within this book is more than just a collection of dietary recommendations; it is a testament to the potential we each possess to regain control over our health and well-being. We have explored the depths of oxalate science, unmasked their presence in everyday foods, and equipped you with the tools to make healthier, pain-free choices.

As we conclude our journey together, I invite you to carry this newfound knowledge forward. Whether you've grappled with chronic pain, approached this topic with curiosity, or stand as a healthcare professional dedicated to improving the lives of your patients, remember that the power to shape your health and future is within your grasp.

With the understanding of oxalates and the guidance provided in this book, you are now empowered to rewrite your story—one meal at a time. The stories of resilience, triumph, and hope within these pages serve as a reminder that no challenge is insurmountable when armed with knowledge and determination.

So, as you step onto your path toward a healthier, pain-free future, keep the lessons we've uncovered close to heart. Harness the wisdom of oxalates, embrace the array of low oxalate foods, and take charge of your well-being. Our journey may have begun in a cozy cafe, but its destination is a life that is vibrant, pain-free, and entirely of your own making.

May the information shared in "Low Oxalate Food List" be your guiding light, illuminating your path to a life free from the grip of chronic pain. Your story, like those we've encountered along the way, has the potential to be one of resilience, transformation, and renewed hope.

BONUS

10 LOW OXALATE RECIPES

Baked Lemon Herb Chicken

Cooking Time: 35 minutes

Servings: 4

Ingredients:

- 4 boneless, skinless chicken breasts
- 1 lemon zested and juiced.
- 2 cloves garlic, minced.
- 1 teaspoon dried oregano
- 1 teaspoon dried thyme
- Salt and pepper to taste
- 2 tablespoons olive oil

Instructions:

1. Preheat the oven to 375°F (190°C).
2. In a small bowl, mix together the lemon zest, lemon juice, minced garlic, dried oregano, dried thyme, salt, and pepper.
3. Place the chicken breasts in a baking dish and pour the lemon herb mixture over them.
4. Drizzle the olive oil on top.

5. Bake for about 25-30 minutes or until the chicken is cooked through and reaches an internal temperature of 165°F (74°C).

6. Serve with your choice of low oxalate vegetables.

Nutritional Information (per serving):

Calories: 245

Protein: 27g

Fat: 12g

Carbohydrates: 4g

Fiber: 1g

Quinoa and Vegetable Stir-Fry

Cooking Time: 25 minutes

Servings: 4

Ingredients:

- 1 cup quinoa, uncooked
- 2 cups water
- 1 tablespoon olive oil
- 1 small onion, chopped.
- 2 cups low oxalate vegetables (e.g., zucchini, bell peppers, broccoli)
- 2 cloves garlic, minced.
- 1/4 cup low-sodium soy sauce
- 1 tablespoon honey
- 1 teaspoon ginger, grated.
- Salt and pepper to taste

Instructions:

1. Rinse quinoa under cold water, then combine with 2 cups of water in a saucepan. Bring to a boil, reduce heat, cover, and simmer for 15 minutes or until the water is absorbed.
2. In a large skillet, heat olive oil over medium heat. Add the chopped onion and stir-fry until translucent.

3. Add your choice of low oxalate vegetables and minced garlic. Stir-fry for about 5-7 minutes until tender-crisp.

4. In a small bowl, whisk together soy sauce, honey, ginger, salt, and pepper.

5. Pour the sauce over the cooked quinoa and stir in the stir-fried vegetables.

6. Serve hot.

Nutritional Information (per serving):

Calories: 280

Protein: 6g

Fat: 5g

Carbohydrates: 51g

Fiber: 5g

(Note: Vegetable selection can affect oxalate content. Choose low oxalate options.)

Grilled Lemon Garlic Shrimp

Cooking Time: 10 minutes

Servings: 4

Ingredients:

- 1-pound large shrimp, peeled and deveined
- Zest and juice of 1 lemon
- 3 cloves garlic, minced.
- 2 tablespoons olive oil
- 1 teaspoon dried basil
- Salt and pepper to taste
- Skewers (if using wooden skewers, soak in water for 30 minutes)

Instructions:

1. In a bowl, combine lemon zest, lemon juice, minced garlic, olive oil, dried basil, salt, and pepper.
2. Thread shrimp onto skewers, then brush with the lemon garlic marinade.
3. Preheat the grill to medium-high heat and lightly oil the grates.
4. Grill shrimp for about 2-3 minutes per side or until they turn pink and opaque.
5. Serve with a side of steamed low oxalate vegetables.

Nutritional Information (per serving):

Calories: 168

Protein: 23g

Fat: 7g

Carbohydrates: 3g

Fiber: 0g

Cilantro-Lime Grilled Chicken

Cooking Time: 20 minutes

Servings: 4

Ingredients:

- 4 boneless, skinless chicken breasts
- Zest and juice of 2 limes
- 2 cloves garlic, minced.
- 1/4 cup fresh cilantro, chopped.
- 2 tablespoons olive oil
- Salt and pepper to taste

Instructions:

1. In a bowl, combine lime zest, lime juice, minced garlic, chopped cilantro, olive oil, salt, and pepper.
2. Place the chicken breasts in a resealable plastic bag and pour the marinade over them. Seal the bag and refrigerate for at least 30 minutes.
3. Preheat the grill to medium-high heat and lightly oil the grates.
4. Grill the chicken for about 6-7 minutes per side or until fully cooked (165°F or 74°C internal temperature).
5. Serve with a side salad of low oxalate greens.

Nutritional Information (per serving):

Calories: 221

Protein: 27g

Fat: 11g

Carbohydrates: 1g

Fiber: 0g

Baked Salmon with Dill

Cooking Time: 20 minutes

Servings: 4

Ingredients:

- 4 salmon fillets
- Zest and juice of 1 lemon
- 2 tablespoons fresh dill, chopped.
- 1 tablespoon olive oil
- Salt and pepper to taste

Instructions:

1. Preheat the oven to 375°F (190°C).
2. In a bowl, combine lemon zest, lemon juice, chopped dill, olive oil, salt, and pepper.
3. Place the salmon fillets on a baking sheet lined with parchment paper. Brush the fillets with the dill and lemon mixture.
4. Bake for about 12-15 minutes or until the salmon flakes easily with a fork.
5. Serve with a side of steamed asparagus or other low oxalate vegetables.

Nutritional Information (per serving):

Calories: 290

Protein: 33g

Fat: 16g

Carbohydrates: 2g

Fiber: 1g

Low Oxalate Greek Salad

Preparation Time: 15 minutes

Servings: 4

Ingredients:

- 2 cups cucumber, diced.
- 2 cups tomatoes, diced.
- 1/2 cup red onion finely chopped.
- 1/4 cup Kalamata olives pitted and sliced.
- 1/4 cup feta cheese, crumbled (optional)
- 2 tablespoons fresh oregano, chopped.
- 2 tablespoons extra-virgin olive oil
- 1 tablespoon red wine vinegar
- Salt and pepper to taste

Instructions:

1. In a large bowl, combine diced cucumber, diced tomatoes, chopped red onion, sliced Kalamata olives, and crumbled feta cheese (if using).
2. In a small bowl, whisk together chopped oregano, olive oil, red wine vinegar, salt, and pepper.
3. Drizzle the dressing over the salad and toss to combine.
4. Serve immediately or refrigerate until ready to serve.

Nutritional Information (per serving without feta):

Calories: 84

Protein: 2g

Fat: 7g

Carbohydrates: 6g

Fiber: 2g

(Note: Feta cheese is optional and can be omitted for a lower oxalate content.)

Low Oxalate Vegetable Soup

Cooking Time: 30 minutes

Servings: 6

Ingredients:

- 2 cups low oxalate vegetables (e.g., cauliflower, zucchini, carrots), chopped.
- 1 small onion, chopped.
- 2 cloves garlic, minced.
- 4 cups low-sodium chicken or vegetable broth
- 1 teaspoon dried thyme
- Salt and pepper to taste
- 2 tablespoons olive oil

Instructions:

1. In a large pot, heat olive oil over medium heat. Add chopped onion and minced garlic and sauté until translucent.
2. Add the chopped low oxalate vegetables and sauté for another 5 minutes.
3. Pour in the chicken or vegetable broth and add dried thyme, salt, and pepper.
4. Bring to a boil, reduce heat, cover, and simmer for 20-25 minutes, or until the vegetables are tender.
5. Use an immersion blender to puree the soup until smooth.

6. Serve hot, garnished with fresh herbs if desired.

Nutritional Information (per serving):

Calories: 64

Protein: 2g

Fat: 4g

Carbohydrates: 7g

Fiber: 2g

Turkey and Vegetable Skewers

Cooking Time: 20 minutes

Servings: 4

Ingredients:

- 1 pound turkey breast, cut into cubes.
- 2 cups low oxalate vegetables (e.g., bell peppers, zucchini, cherry tomatoes), cut into chunks.
- 2 tablespoons olive oil
- 2 teaspoons dried rosemary
- Salt and pepper to taste
- Skewers (if using wooden skewers, soak in water for 30 minutes)

Instructions:

1. Preheat the grill to medium-high heat and lightly oil the grates.
2. Thread turkey cubes and vegetable chunks onto skewers, alternating as desired.
3. In a small bowl, combine olive oil, dried rosemary, salt, and pepper.
4. Brush the skewers with the olive oil mixture.
5. Grill for about 10 minutes, turning occasionally, until the turkey is cooked through, and the vegetables are tender.

6. Serve with a side of quinoa or rice.

Nutritional Information (per serving):

Calories: 245

Protein: 27g

Fat: 11g

Carbohydrates: 8g

Fiber: 2g

Roasted Butternut Squash Soup

Cooking Time: 45 minutes

Servings: 6

Ingredients:

- 1 butternut squash, peeled, seeded, and cubed.

- 1 small onion, chopped.

- 2 cloves garlic, minced.

- 2 tablespoons olive oil

- 4 cups low-sodium vegetable broth

- 1/2 teaspoon ground nutmeg

- Salt and pepper to taste

Instructions:

1. Preheat the oven to 400°F (200°C).

2. In a large bowl, toss the butternut squash cubes with 1 tablespoon of olive oil, salt, and pepper.

3. Spread the squash on a baking sheet and roast for 30-35 minutes, or until tender and lightly browned.

Nutritional Information (per serving without feta):

Calories: 84

Protein: 2g

Fat: 7g

Carbohydrates: 6g

Fiber: 2g

(Note: Feta cheese is optional and can be omitted for a lower oxalate content.)

Roasted Red Pepper and Tomato Soup

Cooking Time: 40 minutes

Servings: 4

Ingredients:

- 4 red bell peppers halved, and seeds removed.
- 4 ripe tomatoes, halved.
- 1 small onion, chopped.
- 2 cloves garlic, minced.
- 2 tablespoons olive oil
- 4 cups low-sodium vegetable broth
- 1 teaspoon dried basil
- Salt and pepper to taste

Instructions:

1. Preheat the oven to 400°F (200°C).
2. Place the red pepper halves and tomato halves on a baking sheet, cut side down. Roast for about 20-25 minutes, or until the skins are charred and blistered.
3. Remove it from the oven and let them cool. Once cooled, peel off the skins and discard.
4. In a large pot, heat olive oil over medium heat. Add chopped onion and minced garlic, and sauté until translucent.

5. Add the roasted red peppers, tomatoes, vegetable broth, dried basil, salt, and pepper.

6. Bring to a boil, then reduce heat and simmer for 15-20 minutes.

7. Use an immersion blender to puree the soup until smooth.

8. Serve hot, garnished with fresh basil leaves.

Nutritional Information (per serving):

Calories: 135

Protein: 2g

Fat: 7g

Carbohydrates: 16g

Fiber: 4g